Contents

What is a kidney stone?

A kidney stone is a solid mass formed from substances in the urine. These substances are normally passed in your urine, but they can become highly concentrated and crystalize when there is not enough urine volume. This is typically a result of inadequate daily fluid intake. These stone-forming substances are:

- Calcium.

- Oxalate.

- Uric acid.

- Phosphate.

- Cystine (rare).

- Xanthine (rare).

These and other chemicals are the "waste products" that must exit the body.

Kidney stones usually range in size from as small as a grain of sand or gravel to the size of a chickpea. They can even be as large as golf balls. Smaller stones (those less than the size of a chickpea) can pass through the urinary tract on their own, but can be associated with significant pain. Depending on their size, you may or may not notice these stones. Larger stones can get trapped in the ureters (tubes which drain the urine from the kidney into the bladder). When this happens, the stones keep urine from exiting the body.

Blocking the flow of urine causes severe pain or bleeding. Stones that can't pass on their own are treated with surgery. This decision is based on the stone size, number of stones/overall amount, locations, and other factors such as shape, type, and patient preference.

What are the most common types of kidney stones?

The most common type of kidney stone is a calcium oxalate stone. This type of stone happens when calcium and oxalate join in your urine. It can happen when you have high quantities of oxalate, low amounts of calcium and aren't drinking enough fluids.

Stones caused by uric acid are also fairly common. These come from a natural substance called purine, which is the byproduct of animal proteins (meat, chicken and fish).

These types of kidney stone run in families, so talk to your healthcare provider about your family history.

How does a kidney stone pass through my urinary tract?

A kidney stone starts out in your kidney. It can stay there and build up for years. Some people may even have kidney stones in their kidney for long period of time without knowing it's there. Once it leaves the kidney, the stone travels down the ureters towards the bladder. The kidney stone enters the bladder and then exits the body through the urethra. Small stones pass out of the body with your urine. Larger stones can get stuck along the way out of the body and may need treatment by your healthcare provider.

How long does it take to form a kidney stone?

You can actually have a kidney stone for years without knowing it's there. Stones can slowly form over years. As long as these stones stay in place within the kidney, you won't feel anything. Pain from a kidney stone typically starts as the stone moves out of the kidney to pass out of the body. Sometimes, a stone can form more quickly — in a few months. This is related to your risk factors and history of kidney stones. Your healthcare provider will discuss all of your risk factors and might do a 24-hour urine test to check how quickly you develop stones.

If I have multiple kidney stones, are they all made of the same substances?

Not all kidney stones are made of the same substances. The materials that make up a kidney stone can vary. You could develop a calcium oxalate stone once and then one made of uric acid another time. This change can happen throughout your life and can be due to things like the treatment you were given for your last stone or other medical conditions.

Who is most likely to experience kidney stones?

Caucasian men in their 30s and 40s have the highest incidence of kidney stones. However, anyone can develop kidney stones.

What are the risk factors for developing kidney stones?

Risks for developing kidney stones include:

There are several risk factors for developing kidney stones. These risks can include:

• Not drinking enough liquids.

• Having a diets that leads to increased excretion of any of the substances listed above.Having a family history of kidney stones.

• Having a blockage in the urinary tract.

Certain medical conditions can also increase your risk of developing a stone because you have higher or lower levels of the substances that make up a kidney stone. These conditions can include:

- Hypercalciuria (high calcium levels in the urine).

- High blood pressure.

- Diabetes.

- Obesity.

- Osteoporosis.

- Gout.

- Kidney cysts.

- Cystic fibrosis.

- Parathyroid disease.

- Inflammatory bowel disease.

- Chronic diarrhea.

- Some surgical procedures, including weight loss surgery or other stomach/intestine surgeries.

There are medications that can increase your risk of developing a stone. These medications can include:

- Diuretics ("water pills").

- Calcium-based antacids.

- Crixivan® (used to treat HIV infections).

- Topamax® and Dilantin® (used to treat seizures).

- Cipro® (ciprofloxacin).

- Ceftriaxone (antibiotics).

Certain foods can also place you at risk of a kidney stone. These foods include:

- Meats and poultry (foods high in animal proteins).

- Sodium (diets high in salt).

- Sugars (fructose, sucrose and corn syrup).

What are the signs and symptoms of kidney stones?

You can actually have a kidney stone in your kidney for years and not know it's there. However, when it starts to move or becomes very large, you may start to feel a few symptoms. Symptoms of a kidney stone can include:

- Feeling pain in the lower back or side of body. This pain can start as a dull ache that may come and go. It can become severe and result in a trip to the emergency room.

- Having nausea and/or vomiting with the pain.

- Seeing blood in the urine.

- Feeling pain when urinating.

- Not being able to urinate.

- Feeling the need to urinate more often.

- Experiencing fever/chills.

- Having urine that smells bad or looks cloudy.

Smaller kidney stones may not cause pain or other symptoms. These small stones pass out of the body in your urine.

DIAGNOSIS AND TESTS

How are kidney stones diagnosed?

Diagnosis of kidney stones starts with a physical exam and review of your medical history. Other tests include:

• Imaging tests: To see the size, shape and location of the stones. These tests determine the most suitable treatment, and sometimes are used to review the result of your treatment. Types of imaging tests used are X-rays, CT scan and ultrasound. Both X-ray tests and CT scans use a small amount of radiation to create their images.

• Blood test: To measure how well your kidneys are functioning, to look for signs of infection, and to look for biochemical problems that lead to forming kidney stones.

- Urine sample test: To look for signs of an infection and to examine the levels of the stone-forming substances — calcium, oxalate, urate, cystine, xanthine and phosphate.

A CT scan of the abdomen is an imaging test that creates a three-dimensional view of the organs within the abdominal cavity. Typically no contrast (or dye) is used for kidney stone diagnosis.. This test shows the stone size and location and conditions that may have caused the stone to form. In addition, the other organs within this area of the body can be evaluated.

An ultrasound of the urinary tract uses sound waves to detect kidney stones and indirect signs of kidney stones, such as changes in the kidney's size and shape.

MANAGEMENT AND TREATMENT

Kidney stone treatment options

How are kidney stones treated?

Your treatment options for a kidney stone can vary on the size of the stone and where it is located in your urinary tract. Treatment options include:

• No treatment: Small stones may not need treatment if they can pass out of the body on their own or if they are not causing a blockage

• Medications: To relax the ureter to allow stones to pass.

• Minimally-invasive procedures: Procedure carried out by entering the body through a small incision in the skin or through the body's natural openings.

No treatment. Sometimes kidney stones can pass through urine on their own depending on the size and location. Drinking plenty of liquids helps the kidney stones travel through the urinary tract. Passing the stone may take up to three weeks.

Medications. Severe pain, requiring an emergency room visit, can be managed with IV narcotics, IV anti-inflammatory drugs, and IV drugs to manage nausea/vomiting. Stones causing less pain can be managed with an anti-inflammatory drug such as ibuprofen. (Caution: Ask your doctor before taking ibuprofen. This drug can increase the risk of kidney failure if taken while having an acute attack of kidney stones – especially in those who have a history of kidney disease and associated illnesses such as diabetes, hypertension and obesity.) Other medications may be given to relax the ureter such as tamsulosin (Flomax®) or nifedipine (Adamant®, Procardia®) so that the stones can pass on their own.

Procedures. There are three types of minimally invasive surgery – ureteroscopy, shockwave lithotripsy and percutaneous nephrolithotomy.

• Ureteroscopy: To perform this procedure, a small instrument, called an ureteroscope, is inserted in the urethra, through the bladder, and into the ureter. This instrument allows stones to be seen and then retrieved in a surgical "basket" or broken apart using a laser. These smaller pieces of kidney stones are then more easily able to exit the body through the urinary tract.

- Shockwave lithotripsy: In this procedure, the patient is placed on a special type of surgical table or tub. High-energy shock waves are sent through water to the stone(s) location. The shock waves break apart the stones, which are then more easily able exit the body through the urinary tract.

- Percutaneous nephrolithotomy: When kidney stones can't be treated by the other procedures – either because there are too many stones, the stones are too large or heavy, or because of their location — percutaneous nephrolithotomy is considered. In this procedure, a tube is inserted directly into the kidney through a small incision made in your back. Stones are then disintegrated by an ultrasound probe and suctioned out so that you do not have to pass any fragments. A urethral stent is placed after the procedure (an internal tube from the kidney to the bladder which is removed one week after surgery in the office). Patients are typically kept overnight for observation and discharged home in the morning.

• Open stone surgery: Open stone surgery, is rarely performed. It is currently only done in 0.3% to 0.7% of cases.

How long does it take to pass a kidney stone?

The amount of time it can take to pass a kidney stone varies. A stone that's smaller than 4 mm may pass within one to two weeks. A stone that's larger than 4 mm could take about two to three weeks to completely pass.

Once the stone reaches the bladder, the stone typically passes within a few days, but may take longer, especially in an older gentleman with a large prostate. However, pain may subside even if the stone is still in the ureter, so it is important to follow up with imaging if you do not pass the stone within 4-6 weeks.

Does cranberry juice help with kidney stones?

Though cranberry juice can help prevent urinary tract infections (UTIs), it doesn't help kidney stones.

Does apple cider vinegar help with kidney stones?

Vinegar is acidic and it can sometimes create changes to your urine which helps stones. However, this doesn't always help. Talk to your healthcare provider about the use of vinegar for kidney stones.

Does lemon juice help with kidney stones?

Lemon juice is rich is citrate, which can help prevent kidney stones from forming. Citrates are found in several citrus fruits, including:

- Lemons.

- Limes.

- Oranges.

- Melons.

PREVENTION

How can kidney stones be prevented?

There are several ways to decrease your risk of kidney stones, including:

• Drinking more fluids, especially water. You should drink at least 64 ounces of liquids per day. Liquids help you stay hydrated. Staying hydrated helps you urinate more often, which helps "flush away" the buildup of the substances that cause kidney stones. If you sweat a lot from your activities, be sure to drink more water.

• Limiting the amount of salt (sodium) in your diet — the DASH diet might be recommended as a low-sodium option.

• Losing weight if you are overweight.

• Limiting the types of foods and drinks that led to the development of your specific type of kidney stone. You may be asked to collect your urine over a 24-hour period. Stone fragments and minerals in the urine can help identify what may have caused your kidney stone. Based on the stone's content, another healthcare professional, a dietitian, can suggest changes in your diet to help decrease your risk of developing more stones.

• Taking medication prescribed by your doctor to help prevent kidney stones based on your specific stone type and any health problems that make you more likely to form a stone.

Should I cut calcium out of my diet if I develop calcium oxalate kidney stones?

If you develop kidney stones composed of calcium, you may be tempted to cut calcium out of your diet. However, this is actually the opposite of what you should do. If you have calcium oxalate stones, the most common type, it's recommended that you have a diet higher in calcium and lower in oxalate. Foods that are high in oxalates include:

• Spinach.

• Rhubarb.

• Strawberries.

• Tea.

• Dried peas and beans.

• Nuts and nut butters.

• Wheat bran.

Foods that are high in calcium include:

- Cow's milk.

- Yogurt.

- Cheese.

- Broccoli.

- Kale.

- Calcium-fortified juices.

- Dried beans.

- Salmon.

- Calcium-fortified hot cereal.

It's also important to drink plenty of fluids to dilute to dilute the substances in your urine.

What other things can I eat or drink to prevent kidney stones?

There are certain foods and drinks might help prevent kidney stones from developing. These can include:

- Drinking plenty of fluids.

- Cutting back on your sodium.

- Increasing the amount of citrates you consume (lemon, lime, orange and melons all have citrates).

- Limiting the amount of oxalates you consume (these are found in foods like spinach, rhubarb, nuts and tea).

Talk to your healthcare provider about the best foods and drinks to prevent the development of future stones. Often, there will be certain foods that work for you but not for another person.

Should I drink soda and coffee if I have kidney stones?

There are some beverages that aren't recommended if you have kidney stones, including soda. Sweetened and dark colas are linked to an increased risk of stone formation. You should also avoid drinks with sugar or corn fructose syrup.

However, coffee has been linked to a decreased risk of developing kidney stones. Studies have shown that people who drink coffee have fewer kidney stones.

OUTLOOK / PROGNOSIS

What is the outlook for kidney stones?

The outlook for kidney stones is very positive, although this is a risk of recurrence (the stones coming back). Many kidney stones pass on their own over time without needing treatment from your healthcare provider. Medications and surgical treatments to remove larger kidney stones are generally very successful and involve little recovery time.

It is possible to get kidney stones multiple times throughout your life. If you find you keep developing kidney stones, your healthcare provider may work with you to discover why the stones happen. Once the cause is found, you may be able to make lifestyle changes to prevent future stones from forming.

Can a large kidney stone cause an injury?

Your risk of injury from a kidney stone can go up based on the size and location of the stone. The size of the stone is important as it passes out of your body. A larger stone could get stuck in your ureter, causing pressure to build up. This can lead to renal failure and, in the worst case (but rare) scenario, you could lose your kidney. The chance of passing a 1 cm stone is less than 10%, and stones larger than 1 cm typically do not pass

How long does pain last after you pass a kidney stone?

Pain from a kidney stone can persist for a few days after completely passing a stone, and this can vary. If the pain persists beyond a week after passing a stone, repeat imaging (typically an ultrasound) is obtained to see if any further blockage is present (sometime due to a remaining stone fragment).

What is the kidney stone diet?

People who wish to prevent kidney stones developing for the first time or reduce the risk of recurrence if they have already had stones should follow these main steps:

- drink plenty of water

- limit their intake of salt and animal protein

- restrict foods that contain high levels of oxalates

- get enough calcium

There is no single diet plan for all types of kidney stones, as they can form due to a buildup of several different minerals in the body. However, many dietitians and doctors who specialize in kidney diseases, or nephrologists, recommend the Dietary Approaches to Stop Hypertension (DASH) diet for people with kidney stones.

This diet has demonstrated the ability to reduce the risk of kidney stone formation and improve other elements of overall health, such as lower blood pressure and a reduced risk of heart disease, stroke, and cancer.

The DASH diet encourages people to consume vegetables, fruits, whole grains, and low-fat dairy. The plan also suggests limiting the intake of salt, sugar, and red meat.

However, dietary changes mainly affect people at risk of the following types of kidney stone:

• calcium oxalate stones

- calcium phosphate stones

- uric acid stones

- cystine stones

People should speak with their healthcare provider to work out which type of kidney stones they have had, if any, to support effective dietary choices. The National Kidney Foundation recommend cutting back on sodium in the diet rather than reducing calcium intake.

Foods to eat

Because kidney stones vary according to the minerals they contain, dietary recommendations will also vary.

A person should talk to their doctor about which foods cause stones to help them determine what they should and should not eat to help avoid the formation of stones in the future.

The following are some suggestions on what to include in a diet to avoid the formation of kidney stones.

Water

Including extra water in the diet can help prevent kidney stones, as they often occur due to dehydration. The National Institute for Diabetes and Digestive and Kidney Diseases (NIDDK) recommend drinking 6–8 glasses every day.

Drinking some other fluids as well as water is acceptable. However, it is important to check sodium levels in the beverage, as many drinks have a high salt content.

It is also best to avoid particularly sugary drinks, such as sweetened juices and sodas.

Calcium and oxalate-rich foods

A person should include foods rich in calcium, especially if they consume many foods that are higher in oxalate, such as spinach. A diet low in calcium increases the risk of developing kidney stones. Calcium and oxalate bind together in the intestines, interrupting the formation of stones.

Some foods to include are:

• low-fat or fat-free milk products

• calcium-fortified foods, such as cereals, bread, and juices

- beans

- calcium-rich vegetables, such as broccoli

- seaweed, such as kelp

Fruits and vegetables

Fruits and vegetables are a necessary part of any diet. Increasing the number of vegetables in their diet can help a person prevent stone formation. Fruits can be dried, frozen, or fresh.

Fruits with high levels of citric acid, such as oranges and lemons, have also demonstrated a positive effect in preventing kidney stones according to a 2014 review of studies.

People should become familiar with fruits and veg that have high oxalate content, including spinach, and try to limit the amount in the diet.

Alternatively, people can combine them with foods that contain high amounts of calcium.

Plant-based protein

Small amounts of animal-based proteins are safe to consume. However, too much animal protein can increase a person's risk of kidney stones.

Dietitians encourage the inclusion of plant-based protein sources in a kidney stone diet. Examples include beans, peas, and lentils.

People should discuss their individual protein needs with a doctor or a dietitian, as the requirement will vary from person to person.

Foods to limit or avoid

Choosing which food to limit depends on the type of stone developing in a person's body.

Foods to limit, include:

- high-sodium foods, including processed, packaged foods as well as meals from fast food establishments

- certain animal proteins, including eggs, fish, and beef

If a person has had calcium oxalate stones, they may wish to restrict their intake of the following foods, which are high oxalate and may increase the risk of recurrence:

- nuts

- peanuts

- spinach

- wheat bran

- rhubarb

Every person is different, and individual needs and dietary requirements will vary.

The most important aspect of managing diet when looking to prevent recurrent kidney stones is speaking to a doctor or dietitian. They will be able to identify the type of kidney stone that is developing and ways to slow or stop its development.

Does the type of kidney stone I had affect food choices I should make?

Yes. If you have already had kidney stones, ask your health care professional which type of kidney stone you had. Based on the type of kidney stone you had, you may be able to prevent kidney stones by making changes in how much sodium, animal protein, calcium, or oxalate is in the food you eat.

You may need to change what you eat and drink for these types of kidney stones:

- Calcium Oxalate Stones

- Calcium Phosphate Stones

- Uric Acid Stones

- Cystine Stones

A dietitian who specializes in kidney stone prevention can help you plan meals to prevent kidney stones. Find a dietitian External link who can help you.

Calcium Oxalate Stones

Reduce oxalate

If you've had calcium oxalate stones, you may want to avoid these foods to help reduce the amount of oxalate in your urine:

- nuts and nut products

- peanuts—which are legumes, not nuts, and are high in oxalate

- rhubarb

- spinach

- wheat bran

Talk with a health care professional about other food sources of oxalate and how much oxalate should be in what you eat.

Reduce sodium

Your chance of developing kidney stones increases when you eat more sodium. Sodium is a part of salt. Sodium is in many canned, packaged, and fast foods. It is also in many condiments, seasonings, and meats.

Talk with a health care professional about how much sodium should be in what you eat. See tips to reduce your sodium intake.

Limit animal protein

Eating animal protein may increase your chances of developing kidney stones.

A health care professional may tell you to limit eating animal protein, including

• beef, chicken, and pork, especially organ meats

• eggs
• fish and shellfish

- milk, cheese, and other dairy products

Although you may need to limit how much animal protein you eat each day, you still need to make sure you get enough protein. Consider replacing some of the meat and animal protein you would typically eat with beans, dried peas, and lentils, which are plant-based foods that are high in protein and low in oxalate.

Talk with a health care professional about how much total protein you should eat and how much should come from animal or plant-based foods.

Get enough calcium from foods

Even though calcium sounds like it would be the cause of calcium stones, it's not. In the right amounts, calcium can block other substances in the digestive tract that may cause stones. Talk with a health care professional about how much calcium you should eat to help prevent getting more calcium oxalate stones and to support strong bones. It may be best to get calcium from low-oxalate, plant-based foods such as calcium-fortified juices, cereals, breads, some kinds of vegetables, and some types of beans. Ask a dietitian or other health care professional which foods are the best sources of calcium for you.

Calcium Phosphate Stones

Reduce sodium

Your chance of developing kidney stones increases when you eat more sodium. Sodium is a part of salt. Sodium is in many canned, packaged, and fast foods. It is also in many condiments, seasonings, and meats.

Talk with a health care professional about how much sodium should be in what you eat. See tips to reduce your sodium intake.

Limit animal protein

Eating animal protein may increase your chances of developing kidney stones.

A health care professional may tell you to limit eating animal protein, including

- beef, chicken, and pork, especially organ meats

- eggs

- fish and shellfish

- milk, cheese, and other dairy products

Although you may need to limit how much animal protein you have each day, you still need to make sure you get enough protein. Consider replacing some of the meat and animal protein you would typically eat with some of these plant-based foods that are high in protein:

• legumes such as beans, dried peas, lentils, and peanuts

• soy foods, such as soy milk, soy nut butter, and tofu

• nuts and nut products, such as almonds and almond butter, cashews and cashew butter, walnuts, and pistachios

• sunflower seeds

Talk with a health care professional about how much total protein you should eat and how much should come from animal or plant-based foods.

Get enough calcium from foods

Even though calcium sounds like it would be the cause of calcium stones, it's not. In the right amounts, calcium can block other substances in the digestive tract that may lead to stones. Talk with a health care professional about how much calcium you should eat to help prevent getting more calcium phosphate stones and to support strong bones. It may be best to get calcium from plant-based foods such as calcium-fortified juices, cereals, breads, some kinds of vegetables, and some types of beans. Ask a dietitian or other health care professional which foods are the best sources of calcium for you.

Uric Acid Stones

Limit animal protein

Eating animal protein may increase your chances of developing kidney stones.

A health care professional may tell you to limit eating animal protein, including

• beef, chicken, and pork, especially organ meats

• eggs

• fish and shellfish

• milk, cheese, and other dairy products

Although you may need to limit how much animal protein you have each day, you still need to make sure you get enough protein. Consider replacing some of the meat and animal protein you would typically eat with some of these plant-based foods that are high in protein:

- legumes such as beans, dried peas, lentils, and peanuts

- soy foods, such as soy milk, soy nut butter, and tofu

- nuts and nut products, such as almonds and almond butter, cashews and cashew butter, walnuts, and pistachios

- sunflower seeds

Talk with a health care professional about how much total protein you should eat and how much should come from animal or plant-based foods.

Losing weight if you are overweight is especially important for people who have had uric acid stones.

Cystine Stones

Drinking enough liquid, mainly water, is the most important lifestyle change you can make to prevent cystine stones. Talk with a health care professional about how much liquid you should drink.

Tips to Reduce Your Sodium Intake

Most Americans consume too much sodium. Adults should aim to consume less than 2,300 mg a day External link.3 One teaspoon of table salt has 2,325 milligrams (mg) of sodium. If you have had calcium oxalate or calcium phosphate stones, you should follow this guideline, even if you take medicine to prevent kidney stones.

Here are some tips to help you reduce your sodium intake:

- Check the Percent Daily Value (%DV) for sodium on the Nutrition Facts label found on many foods. Low in sodium is 5% or less, and high in sodium is 20% or more.

- Consider writing down how much sodium you consume each day.

- When eating out, ask about the sodium content in the food.

- Cook from scratch. Avoid processed and fast foods, canned soups and vegetables, and lunch meats.

- Look for foods labeled: sodium free, salt free, very low sodium, low sodium, reduced or less sodium, light in sodium, no salt added, unsalted, and lightly salted.

Check labels for ingredients and hidden sodium, such as

- sodium bicarbonate, the chemical name for baking soda

- baking powder, which contains sodium bicarbonate and other chemicals

- disodium phosphate

- monosodium glutamate, or MSG

- sodium alginate

- sodium nitrate or nitrite

Will it help or hurt to take a vitamin or mineral supplement?

The B vitamins which include thiamine, riboflavin, niacin, B6 and B12 have not been shown to be harmful to people with kidney stones. In fact, some studies have shown that B6 may actually help people with high urine oxalate. However, it is best to check with your healthcare professional or dietitian for advice on the use of vitamin C, vitamin D, fish liver oils or other mineral supplements containing calcium since some supplements can increase the chances of stone formation in some individuals.

Is there anything else to do to help prevent kidney stones?

1. It's Not "One and Done." Passing a kidney stone is often described as one of the most painful experiences an individual will experience. Unfortunately, it's not always a one-time event. Take action NOW! Without the right medicines,

diet, and fluid intake, stones can come back. Returning kidney stones could also mean there are other problems, including kidney disease.

2. When Life Hands You Kidney Stones… don't worry.

And as the saying goes, "make lemonade." It's important to consider dietary remedies alongside prescription medications.

Next time you drive past a lemonade stand, consider your kidneys. Chronic kidney stones are often treated with an alkali (less acidic) citrate, such as potassium citrate to help prevent certain stones if urine citrate is low and urine pH levels are too low (or too acidic). Citrus juices do contain citrate (citric acid), but large amounts might be needed. Also, be careful of sugar.

Lemon juice concentrate (4 oz per day) mixed with water can be considered. Alkali citrate can be prescribed and is available over-the-counter. Alkali citrate can be given with a mineral(s), such as sodium, potassium or magnesium to help prevent stone formation. The aim is to increase urine citrate (for prevention of calcium stones) and increase urine pH (or make urine less acidic or more alkaline, for prevention of uric acid and cystine stones). The goal is to keep pH in balance. Speak with a doctor or other healthcare professional about which treatment options are right for you, including over-the-counter products and home remedies. People with kidney disease may need to watch their intake of sodium, potassium or other minerals, depending on the stage of kidney disease or other factors.

Diet Recommendations for Kidney Stones

General Recommendations

1. Drink plenty of fluid: 2-3 quarts/day

o This includes any type of fluid such as water, coffee and lemonade which have been shown to have a beneficial effect with the exception of grapefruit juice and soda.

o This will help produce less concentrated urine and ensure a good urine volume of at least 2.5L/day

2. Limit foods with high oxalate content

o Spinach, many berries, chocolate, wheat bran, nuts, beets, tea and rhubarb should be eliminated from your diet intake

3. Eat enough dietary calcium

o Three servings of dairy per day will help lower the risk of calcium stone formation. Eat with meals.

4. Avoid extra calcium supplements

o Calcium supplements should be individualized by your physician and registered kidney dietitian

5. Eat a moderate amount of protein

o High protein intakes will cause the kidneys to excrete more calcium therefore this may cause more stones to form in the kidney

6. Avoid high salt intake

o High sodium intake increases calcium in the urine which increases the chances of developing stones

o Low salt diet is also important to control blood pressure.

7. Avoid high doses of vitamin C supplements

o It is recommend to take 60mg/day of vitamin C based on the US Dietary Reference Intake

o Excess amounts of 1000mg/day or more may produce more oxalate in the body

How does the diet work?

Some foods contain certain chemicals or compounds that can influence the production of kidney stones, particularly if a person regularly eats them in high amounts.

By limiting the intake of these foods, the risk of kidney stones reduces.

Can diet alone treat kidney stones?

For some people, dietary changes may be enough to prevent kidney stones from occurring.

In other cases, additional treatment may be necessary, including medication to break the stones up or surgery to remove the stones.

If stones become extremely painful, it is best to seek consultation with a doctor or nephrologist so they can recommend the best course of action.

Do any herbal supplements help reduce the risk of kidney stones?

People have used many herbs throughout time. Traditionally, people have used apple cider vinegar to prevent and treat kidney stones, and studies in the lab have shown that it can reduce the development of stones.

According to one cross-sectional study, the acetic acid in apple cider vinegar reduces pain and inflammation.

People have also used wheatgrass for centuries to improve health and because it contains certain compounds that cause increased urine output, reducing the risk that kidney stones will develop.

KIDNEY STONE DIET RECIPES

In this part are nourishing kidney stone diet recipes to keep your kidney stone at bay.

Nats' Ground Chicken and Veggie Mix-Up

Preparation time

25 minutes

Ingredients:

• 1 pound of ground chicken (or any protein you like).

• Variety of low oxalate veggies (look at your oxalate list to choose what you want and LIKE).

Instructions

1. Add olive oil to a medium saute pan and heat on medium-high heat.

2. When the oil is shimmering, add 1 chopped onion (you can also add some garlic, I can't tolerate garlic so I skip it).

3. In another saute pan, put oil in the pan and cook ground chicken (or whatever protein you have chosen).

4. Chop and add your other low oxalate veggies to the pan with the onions.

5. When your vegetables are cooked add whatever herbs or spices you want.

6. After your chicken is done, add veggie mix and you are done! So simple and so good.

Southwest Baked Egg Breakfast Cups

Preparation time

25 minutes

Ingredients

- 3 cups rice, cooked

- 4 ounces cheddar cheese, shredded

- 4 ounces green chilies, diced

- 2 ounces pimentos, drained and diced

- ½ cup skim milk

- 2 eggs, beaten

- ½ teaspoon ground cumin

- ½ teaspoon black pepper

- nonstick cooking spray

Instructions

1. In a large bowl, combine rice, 2 ounces of cheese, chilies, pimentos, milk, eggs, cumin and pepper.

2. Spray muffin cups with nonstick cooking spray.

3. Spoon mixture evenly into 12 muffin cups.

4. Sprinkle top of each cup with the remaining 2 ounces of shredded cheese.

5. Bake at 400° F for 15 minutes or until set.

Blueberry Muffins

Preparation time

45 minutes

Ingredients

- ½ cup unsalted butter

- 1 ¼ cups sugar

- 2 eggs

- 2 cups 1% milk

- 2 cups all-purpose flour

- 2 teaspoons baking powder

- ½ teaspoon salt

- 2 ½ cups fresh blueberries

- 2 teaspoons sugar (for topping)

Instructions

1. Using a mixer set on low speed, blend margarine and sugar until creamy and fluffy.

2. Add eggs one at a time and mix until blended.

3. Sift dry ingredients and add alternately with milk.

4. Mash ½ cup blueberries and stir in by hand. Then add remaining blueberries and stir in by hand.

5. Spray muffin cups and surface of pan with vegetable oil. Place muffins cups in tin.

6. Pile muffin mixture high in each muffin cup. Sprinkle sugar over muffin tops.

7. Bake at 375° F for 25–30 minutes. Cool in pan for at least 30 minutes before removing carefully.

Easy Turkey Breakfast Burritos

Preparation time

30 minutes

Ingredients

- 1 pound of ground turkey or use 1 pound leftover turkey meatloaf, cubed small

- 8 6-inch flour burrito shells

- ¼ cup canola oil

- 8 beaten eggs, scrambled

- ¼ cup diced onions

- ¼ cup fresh bell peppers (red, yellow or green), diced

- 2 tablespoons seeded jalapeño peppers

- 2 tablespoons fresh scallions, chopped

- 2 tablespoons fresh cilantro, chopped

- ½ teaspoon chili powder

- ½ teaspoon smoked paprika

- 1 cup shredded Monterey Jack and Cheddar cheese

Instructions

1. Sauté meatloaf, onions, peppers, scallions and cilantro in half the oil until translucent.

2. Stir in spices and then turn off heat.

3. Using another large sauté pan, set pan to medium-high heat and add in remaining oil and scrambled eggs.

4. Place equal amounts of vegetable and meatloaf mix, cheese and eggs in burrito shells, then fold and serve.

Spicy Tofu Scrambler

Preparation time

35 minutes

Ingredients

- 1 teaspoon olive oil

- ¼ cup red bell pepper, chopped

- ¼ cup green bell pepper, chopped

- 1 cup firm tofu (choose less than 10% calcium)

- 1 teaspoon onion powder

- ¼ teaspoon garlic powder

- 1 clove garlic, minced

- ⅛ teaspoon turmeric

Instructions

1. In a medium-sized, nonstick skillet, sauté garlic and both bell peppers in olive oil.

2. Rinse and drain tofu and crumble it into the skillet.

3. Add the remaining ingredients.

4. Stir and cook on low to medium heat until the tofu turns a slight golden brown, about 20 minutes.

5. Water will evaporate out of the mixture.

6. Serve tofu scrambler warm.

Chocolate Pancakes With Moon Pie Stuffing

Preparation time

30 minutes

Ingredients

Moon Pie Stuffing:

- 1 tablespoon unsweetened cocoa powder

- ¼ cup heavy cream

- ½ cup cream cheese, softened

- ½ cup marshmallow cream

Chocolate Pancakes:

- 1 cup flour

- 3 tablespoons sugar

- 3 tablespoons unsweetened cocoa powder

- ½ teaspoon baking soda

- 1 tablespoon lemon juice

- 1 egg

- 1 cup 2% milk

- 2 tablespoons canola oil

- 2 teaspoons vanilla extract

- 2/3 cup Body Fortress® vanilla whey protein powder

Instructions

Moon Pie Filling:

1. Beat cocoa and heavy cream together until stiff peaks are formed.

2. Whip in cream cheese, marshmallow cream and whey protein powder for about a minute or until well blended, but don't overbeat.

3. Cover and set aside in fridge.

Pancakes:

1. Mix all the dry ingredients together in a large bowl and set aside.

2. Mix all the wet ingredients in medium-size bowl.

3. Slowly fold in wet ingredients to the dry ingredients just until wet, but don't over mix.

4. Cook the pancakes on a lightly oiled griddle on medium heat or 375° F.

5. Use about 1/8 cup of batter to form 4-inch pancakes, flipping when they start to bubble

Fluffy Homemade Buttermilk Pancakes

Preparation time

20 minutes

Ingredients

- 2 cups all-purpose flour

- 1 teaspoon cream of tartar

- 1½ teaspoons baking soda

- 2 tablespoons sugar

- 2 cups low-fat buttermilk

- 2 large eggs

- ¼ cup canola oil and 1 tablespoon canola oil (for cooking)

Instructions

Warm up a skillet on medium heat.

1. Combine dry ingredients in a large bowl.

2. Add dry ingredients to buttermilk, oil and egg mixture.

3. Use a whisk or spoon to blend the dry ingredients until they are completely moist.

4. Use a tablespoon of canola oil to grease the skillet.

5. Using a ⅓-cup measuring cup, scoop the pancake mixture on the skillet. Each pancake should spread to about 4 inches across.

6. Leave about 2" between the pancakes for easy flipping.

7. Flip pancakes using a spatula—do this when the bubbles on the top of the pancakes have

mostly disappeared. Allow the other side to brown until the center no longer appears wet.

8. Move to serving dish.

Lemon Orzo Spring Salad

Preparation time

30 minutes

Ingredients

- ¾ cup or ¼ box orzo pasta

- ¼ cup fresh yellow peppers, diced

- ¼ cup fresh red peppers, diced

- ¼ cup fresh green peppers, diced

- ½ cup fresh red or Vidalia onion, diced

- 2 cups fresh zucchini, medium-cubed

- ¼ cup and 2 tablespoons olive oil

- 3 tablespoons fresh lemon juice

- 1 teaspoon lemon zest

- 3 tablespoons grated Parmesan cheese

- 2 tablespoons fresh rosemary, chopped

- ½ teaspoon black pepper

- ½ teaspoon dried oregano

- ½ teaspoon red pepper flakes

Instructions

1. Cook orzo pasta according to box directions, drain and let sit. (Do not rinse.)

2. Sauté peppers, onions and zucchini on medium-high heat with 2 tablespoons of oil in large pan until translucent.

3. Mix lemon juice, lemon zest, ¼ cup olive oil, cheese, rosemary, pepper, oregano and red pepper flakes in a large bowl.

4. Add sautéed vegetables and orzo pasta into the large bowl and fold gently until well mixed.

5. Chill or serve at room temperature

Chilled Veggie and Shrimp Noodle Salad

Preparation time

15 minutes

Ingredients

- 1 pound package of dry Spaghetti, noodles cooked and chilled (don't rinse)

- 4 cups cooked cocktail shrimp, peeled, deveined, tailless and cut in half; or 14-ounce pack of cooked salad shrimp

- 1 cup fresh scallions, sliced on the bias

- 2 cups fresh broccoli florets

- 1 cup fresh carrots, shredded

- 2 cups fresh shitake mushrooms, chopped

- 2 tablespoons sesame oil

- 2 teaspoons chili oil

- ½ cup rice wine vinegar

- 2 tablespoons fresh garlic, chopped

- 1 tablespoon fresh ginger, chopped

- ¼ cup low-sodium soy sauce substitute (recipe below)

- ¼ cup fresh lime juice (about 2 limes) and zest of 1 lime (1 tablespoon)

- Low-Sodium Soy Sauce Substitute (makes 1 cup):

- 4 teaspoons Better Than Bouillon®

- Chicken Base (low sodium)

- 1 teaspoon reduced-sodium soy sauce

- 4 teaspoons balsamic vinegar

- 2 teaspoons dark molasses

- ¼ teaspoon ground ginger

- ¼ teaspoon white pepper

- ¼ teaspoon garlic powder

- 1½ cups water

Instructions

1. Combine ingredients for soy sauce substitute in small saucepan.

2. Stir on medium heat. Allow to reduce and thicken slightly to about 1 cup. Store remainder in refrigerator.

3. Then, mix first 6 ingredients together in large bowl and set aside.

4. Blend remaining ingredients together in blender until well incorporated, about 1 minute.

5. Pour dressing mixture over pasta mixture. Toss until well coated, then serve.

Knock-Your-Socks-Off Chicken Broccoli Stromboli

Preparation time

35 minutes

Ingredients

- 1 pound store-bought pizza dough (Note: dough can be purchased at some local pizzerias as well as grocery stores)

- 2 cups fresh broccoli florets, blanched

- 2 cups diced cooked chicken breast

- 1 cup shredded low-salt mozzarella cheese

- 1 tablespoon fresh garlic, chopped

- 1 tablespoon fresh oregano, chopped

- 1 teaspoon crushed red pepper flakes

- 2 tablespoons flour

- 2 tablespoons olive oil

Instructions

1. Preheat oven to 400° F.

2. Mix chicken, cheese, pepper flakes, broccoli, garlic and oregano in large bowl and set aside.

3. Dust tabletop with flour and roll out dough until you reach an 11" x 14" rectangular shape.

4. Place chicken mixture about 2 inches from the edge of the dough, along the longest side.

5. Roll and pinch the ends and seam until tightly sealed (a fork can be used to crimp edges for a tight seal).

6. Brush the top with olive oil and make 3 small slits on the top of the dough.

7. Bake 8–12 minutes or until golden brown on lightly oiled baking sheet tray.

8. Remove, let sit for 3–5 minutes, then slice and serve

Cool and Crispy Cucumber Salad

Preparation time

Ingredients

- 2 cups fresh cucumber (sliced into ¼-inch slices, peeling is optional)

- 2 tablespoons Italian or Caesar salad dressing

- Fresh ground black pepper to taste

Instructions

1. In medium-size bowl with lid, combine cucumber and salad dressing.

2. Cover with lid, shake to coat.

3. Sprinkle with ground black pepper.

4. Refrigerate.

5. Best served cold.

Smoky & Savory Salmon Dip

Preparation time

1 hour 15 minutes

Ingredients

- 1 pound fresh skinless, boneless salmon cut into 4 pieces

- 2 teaspoons smoked paprika

- 1 cup cream cheese

- ¼ cup capers

- ¼ cup lemon juice and zest of half a lemon (about 1 teaspoon)

- 2 tablespoons red onions, finely diced

- 1 teaspoon ground black pepper

- 1 tablespoon fresh parsley, chopped

Instructions

1. Poach the salmon in 2 cups of water and 1 teaspoon of smoked paprika for 4–6 minutes on medium-high heat; the pot should be covered but it should not reach a boil.

2. Remove and chill for at least 30 minutes.

3. Mix all of the other ingredients together until smooth.

4. Break salmon into bite-sized pieces and fold into the cream cheese mixture.

5. Chill salmon dip for 20–30 minutes. Serve with celery sticks, corn chips and carrots or rolled in a leaf of iceberg lettuce.

Herb-Roasted Chicken Breasts

Preparation time

5 hours

Ingredients

• 1 pound boneless, skinless chicken breasts

• 1 medium onion

• 1–2 garlic cloves

• 2 tablespoons Mrs. Dash® Garlic and Herb Seasoning Blend

• 1 teaspoon ground black pepper

• ¼ cup olive oil

Instructions

Marinating:

1. Chop onion and garlic and place in a bowl. Add Mrs. Dash Seasoning, ground pepper and olive oil.

2. Add chicken breasts to the marinade, cover it, then refrigerate for at least 4 hours or overnight.

Baking:

1. Preheat the oven to 350°F.

2. Cover a baking sheet with foil, place the marinated chicken breasts on the pan.

3. Pour the remaining marinade over the chicken and bake at 350°F for 20 minutes.

4. Broil an additional 5 minutes for browning.

Fired-Up Zucchini Turkey Burger

Preparation time

30 minutes

Ingredients

- 1 pound ground turkey meat

- 1 cup zucchini, shredded

- ½ cup onion, minced

- 1 jalapeño pepper, sliced lengthwise, seeded and minced

- 1 egg

- 1 teaspoon Mrs. Dash® Extra Spicy Blend

- 2 fresh poblano peppers, sliced in half lengthwise and seeded

- 1 teaspoon mustard (optional)

Instructions

1. Mix the first 6 ingredients thoroughly.

2. Form meat mixture into 4 turkey burger patties.

3. Turkey burgers may be grilled outdoors on a grill or on an electric griddle.

4. The peppers can be grilled alongside turkey burgers until the skin is tender and blistered.

5. Grill turkey burgers to an internal temperature of 165° F or until center is no longer pink.

6. Top the patty with sliced grilled peppers and serve on a hamburger bun.

Egg Fried Rice

Preparation time

25 minutes

Ingredients

- 2 teaspoons dark sesame oil

- 2 eggs

- 2 egg whites

- 1 tablespoon canola oil

- 1 cup bean sprouts

- ⅓ cup green onions, chopped

- 4 cups cooked rice, cold

- 1 cup frozen peas, thawed

- ¼ teaspoon ground black pepper

Instructions

1. Combine the sesame oil, eggs and egg whites in a small bowl.

2. Stir well and set aside.

3. Heat canola oil in a large nonstick skillet over medium-high heat.

4. Add egg mixture and stir-fry until done.

5. Add bean sprouts and green onions. Stir-fry for 2 minutes.

6. Add rice and peas. Continue to stir-fry until heated thoroughly.

7. Season with black pepper and serve immediately.

Veggie Egg

Preparation time

30 minutes

INGREDIENTS

- 4 whole eggs

- 1 c cauliflower

- 3 c fresh spinach

- 1 garlic clove, minced

- 1/4 c bell pepper, chopped

- 1/4 cup onion, chopped

- 1/4 tsp black pepper

- 1 tbsp oil of choice (coconut or avocado oil is good for high heat)

- fresh parsley and spring onion for garnish

- optional tomatoes on side if no potassium restriction

INSTRUCTIONS

1. Beat eggs with pepper until light and fluffy, set aside.

2. Heat oil over medium heat in large skillet.

3. Add onions and peppers to skillet and saute until peppers are translucent and golden.

4. Add garlic, stirring quickly to combine and immediately adding cauliflower and spinach.

5. Saute vegetables, turn heat to medium-low and cover for 5 minutes.

6. Add eggs, stirring to combine with vegetables.

7. When the eggs are cooked thoroughly, top with fresh parsley or spring onions.

8. If no potassium restriction can serve with a side of bright fresh tomatoes topped with cracker black pepper.

9. A touch of feta or a strong sharp cheese would also be delicious with these

Shrimp SaladPreparation time

40 minutes

Ingredients

- 1 pound shrimp, boiled, chopped and deveined

- 1 hard boiled egg, chopped

- 1 tablespoon celery, chopped

- 1 tablespoon green pepper, chopped

- 1 tablespoon onion, chopped

- 2 tablespoons mayonnaise

- 1 teaspoon lemon juice

- ½ teaspoon chili powder

- ⅛ teaspoon Tabasco® or hot sauce

- ½ teaspoon dry mustard

- lettuce, chopped or shredded (optional)

Instructions

1. Combine all ingredients except lettuce in a mixing bowl

2. mix well.

3. Chill in refrigerator for 30 minutes.

4. Serve as a salad over a bed of lettuce, if desired, or serve on a sandwich.

Tuna-Nood le Skillet

DinnerPreparation time

Preparation time

Ingredients

• vegetable cooking spray

- 2 tablespoons minced fresh onion

- ⅔ cup water

- ¼ teaspoon curry powder

- ¼ teaspoon black pepper

- 1 10 ¾-ounce can low sodium cream of mushroom soup, undiluted

- 2 cups hot cooked rotini (corkscrew pasta, cooked without salt or fat)

- ½ cup frozen green peas, thawed

- 1 9 ¼-ounce low sodium albacore tuna, with water, drained

- chopped fresh parsley (optional)

Instructions

1. Coat a large non-stick skillet with cooking spray; place over medium heat.

2. Add onion; sauté until tender.

3. Combine water, curry powder, pepper and soup in a bowl; stir well and add to skillet.

4. Add cooked rotini, peas, and tuna; stir well.

5. Cook uncovered, over low heat 10 minutes, stirring occasionally.

6. Sprinkle with parsley, if desired.

Chicken Vegetable SaladPreparation time

10 minutes

Ingredients

* 1 ½ cups cooked chicken, diced

* ½ cup green pepper, finely chopped

* ½ cup celery, finely diced

* ½ cup onions, finely chopped

* 3 tablespoons pimentos, diced

* ½ cup salad dressing or light mayonnaise

* 1 tablespoon lemon juice

Instructions

1. In a large bowl, combine chicken, green pepper, celery, onions and pimentos.

2. In a small bowl, mix mayonnaise and lemon juice.

3. Pour over chicken mixture.

4. Mix well, cover and chill.

5. Serve in a lettuce cups.

Spicy LambPreparation time

8 hours 30 minutes

Ingredients

- ¼ cup vegetable oil

- 1 ½ tablespoons garlic powder

- 3 teaspoons dry mustard

- 1 leg of lamb (trimmed for roasting)

Instructions

1. Blend ingredients for marinade: oil, garlic powder and mustard.

2. Coat leg of lamb with marinade; refrigerate 6-8 hours or overnight.

3. Adjust meat on barbecue spit and roast for 30 minutes per pound or until 170ºF on meat thermometer, basting meat continuously with marinade.

Cream Cheese CookiesPreparation time

1 hour 30 minutes

Ingredients

* 1 cup butter or margarine, softened

* 1 3-ounce package cream cheese, softened

* 1 cup sugar

* 1 egg yolk

* 2 ½ cups all-purpose flour

* 1 teaspoon vanilla extract

* candied cherry halves

Instructions

1. Preheat oven to 325°F.

2. Cream butter and cream cheese; slowly add sugar, beating until fluffy.

3. Beat in egg yolk; add flour and vanilla, mix well.

4. Chill dough at least one hour

5. Shape dough into 1" balls; place on greased cookie sheets.

6. Gently press a cherry half into each cookie.

7. Bake for 12-15 minutes.

Pineapple Pound CakePreparation time

1 hour 10 minutes

Ingredients

for cake

- 3 cups sugar

- 1 ½ cups butter

- 6 whole eggs and 4 egg whites

- 1 teaspoon vanilla extract

- 3 cups all-purpose flour, sifted

- 1 10-ounce can crushed pineapple (drain and reserve juice)

Instructions

1. Preheat oven to 350°F.

2. Beat together sugar and butter until smooth and creamy.

3. Add eggs and egg whites two at a time, mixing after each addition.

4. Add vanilla. Add sifted flour and mix well.

5. Add drained, crushed pineapple.

6. Bake for 45 minutes to 1 hour.

7. In a medium saucepan, mix together ingredients for glaze. Stir frequently. Bring to a boil, until desired thickness is reached. Pour over top of cake while hot.

Whipped Cream Pound CakePreparation time

1 hour 15 minutes

Ingredients

- 2 sticks margarine or butter, softened

- 3 cups sugar

- 6 eggs

- 3 cups cake flour (sift once before measuring)

- ½ pint whipping cream

- 1 teaspoon vanilla flavoring

Instructions

1. Preheat oven to 350°F.

2. Grease and flour tube pan.

3. All ingredients should be at room temperature.

4. Cream margarine and sugar together until fluffy.

5. Add eggs, one at a time, beating after each addition.

6. Gradually add flour and whipping cream, blending between each addition.

7. Beat well for 30 seconds; stir in vanilla flavoring.

8. Pour batter into tube pan; bake for 50-60 minutes.

Fruit Crunch (Crumb Top Pie)Preparation time

45 minutes

Ingredients

- 4 large tart apples, pared, cored and sliced
- ¾ cup sugar

- ½ cups all-purpose flour, sifted

- ⅓ cup margarine, softened

- ¾ cup rolled oats

- ¾ teaspoon nutmeg

Instructions

1. Preheat oven to 375°F.

2. Place apples in a greased 8" square pan. 3. Combine remaining ingredients in a medium bowl, and spread over fruit. 4. Bake 30-35 minutes or until fruit is tender and lightly browned.

Frozen Lemon DessertPreparation time

5 hours 30 minutes

Ingredients

• 4 eggs, separated

• ⅔ cup sugar

• ¼ cup lemon juice1 tablespoon lemon peel, grated

• 1 cup whipping cream, whipped

• 2 cups vanilla wafers (about 40), crushed

Instructions

1. Beat egg yolks until very thick.

2. Gradually beat in sugar, beating well after each addition.

3. Add lemon juice and lemon peel; blend well.

4. Cook in double boiler over hot water stirring constantly until thick.

5. Remove from heat and allow to cool.

6. Beat egg whites until stiff peaks form.

7. Fold egg whites into cooled thickened mixture.

8. Fold in whipped cream

9. Spread 1 ½ cups vanilla wafer crumbs in bottom of freezer tray or 10" x 6" x 1 ½" baking dish.

10. Spoon lemon mixture over crumbs.

11.Top with remaining vanilla wafer crumbs.

12. Freeze until firm, several hours or overnight.

Fruit Salad

Preparation time

5 minutes

Ingredients

- 2 cups canned fruit cocktail, drained

- 1 cup canned pineapple chunks, drained

- 1 cup whole or sliced strawberries, hulled

- 1 cup apple, peeled, cored and diced

- 1 cup marshmallows

- ½ cup non-dairy whipped topping

Instructions

1. Combine all fruits together.

2. Add marshmallows and whipped topping; mix well.

3. Refrigerate and serve chilled.

Chocolate Pie Shell

Preparation time

40 minutes

Ingredients

3 cups cocoa krispies, crushed

½ stick (4 tablespoons) butter

cooking sprayInstructions

1. Place crushed cereal and melted butter in a bowl. Stir well.

2. Spray 9" pie pan with cooking spray.

3. Press mixture into pan.

4. Chill at least 30 minutes before filling.

Strawberry Sorbet

Preparation time

5 minutes

Ingredients

- ¼ cup sugar

- 1 cup frozen or fresh strawberries, cleaned,

- 1 tablespoon lemon juice

- ¼ cup water

- 1 ¼ cups crushed or cubed ice

Instructions

1. Place ice in a blender.

2. Add all other ingredients, turn speed to crush or liquefy.

Cranberry Punch

Preparation time

5 minutes

Ingredients

• 3 quarts cranberry juice

• 3 quarts pineapple juice1 quart lemonade, frozen, undiluted

- 1 quart water

- 3 28-ounce bottles ginger ale

Instructions

1. Mix all ingredients together.

2. Chill and serve.

Russian Tea

Preparation time

5 minutes

Ingredients

- 2 cups Tang½ cup sugar1 dry lemonade mix (2 quart size)1 cup instant tea1 teaspoon cloves1 teaspoon cinnamon

Instructions

1. Combine all ingredients.

2. Store in a covered container.

3. To mix: add one tablespoon to 8-ounces hot water.

4. Serve hot.

Baked Apples with Craisins

Preparation time

1 hour

Ingredients

- 4 apples for baking

- 1 cup apple juice

- ¼ cup brown sugar, packed

- 2 tablespoon Craisins

- red cinnamon candies

Instructions

1. Preheat oven to 375ºF.

2. Wash and core the apples. Set aside.

3. Using a square baking pan (9 "x 9" x 1 ¾"), blend the apple juice and brown sugar.

4. Place apples in pan.

5. Fill apple centers with craisins and cinnamon candies.

6. Place pan in the oven. Spoon juice over apples occasionally during baking to glaze the apples and keep them from drying out. 7. Bake 40 to 45 minutes, or until apples are tender when pierced with a fork.

English Muffin Pizza

Preparation time

15 minutes

Ingredients

- 1 split english muffin

- ¼ cup pizza sauce

- 2 tablespoons shredded mozzarella cheese

Instructions

1. Toast english muffins.

2. Spread pizza sauce evenly on muffin halves.

3. Sprinkle cheese and add toppings.

4. Place the muffin halves on tray and put into toaster oven, set on broil.

5. Broil for about 5 minutes, watching carefully to remove when cheese is golden and melted.

Bourbon-Glazed Skirt Steak

Preparation time

2 hours

Ingredients

Bourbon Glaze:

- ¼ cup diced shallots

- 3 tablespoons unsalted butter, chilled and cubed

- 1 cup bourbon

- ¼ cup dark brown sugar

- 2 tablespoons Dijon mustard

- 1 tablespoon black pepper

Skirt Steak:

- 2 tablespoons grape seed oil

- ½ teaspoon dried oregano

- ½ teaspoon smoked paprika

- 1 teaspoon black pepper

- 1 tablespoon red wine vinegar

- 2 pounds skirt steak

Instructions

Bourbon Glaze:

1. In small saucepan on medium-high heat, brown shallots in 1 tablespoon butter.

2. Reduce heat to low, remove pan from stove, add bourbon and then place saucepan back on stove.

3. Cook for 10–15 minutes, or until reduced by about one third.

4. Add brown sugar, mustard and black pepper and stir until bubbly.

5. Turn off heat and stir in the remaining 2 tablespoons of cold, cubed butter, stirring constantly until well incorporated.

Skirt Steak:

1. Mix first 5 ingredients in gallon-size sealable storage bag, add steaks and shake well.

2. Allow steaks to marinate in bag at room temperature for 30–45 minutes.

3. Remove steaks from bag, grill for 15– 20 minutes each side, then remove and let rest for 10 minutes.

4. Slice and serve with a drizzle of sauce; or leave whole and brush with glaze and put in

preheated broiler for 4–6 minutes, or until desired look.

Pumpkin Strudel

Preparation time

40 minutes

Ingredients

- 1½ cups canned pumpkin, sodium-free, unsweetened

- ⅛ teaspoon grated nutmeg

- 1 teaspoon pure vanilla extract

- 4 tablespoons sugar

- ½ teaspoon ground cinnamon

- ½ stick (4 tablespoons) butter, unsalted, melted

- 12 sheets phyllo dough (follow package directions for defrosting if frozen)

Instructions

1. Position the oven rack in the middle of the oven.

2. Preheat the oven to 375° F.

3. In a medium-sized bowl, combine the canned pumpkin, nutmeg, vanilla extract, 2 tablespoons of sugar and ½ tablespoon of cinnamon until well-mixed.

4. Using a pastry brush, coat the bottom of a nonstick medium sheet tray with the melted butter.

5. On a clean work surface, lay down a single sheet of phyllo dough, and brush it with the butter.

6. Then create a stack of buttered phyllo sheets, brushing every other phyllo sheet with butter. (Be sure to save a little melted butter to brush the top of the rolled filled strudel, so go lightly when brushing in between layers.)

7. Keep remaining phyllo dough sheets covered with plastic wrap until ready for use, so they do not dry out.

8. Once all 12 sheets are used, spoon the mixture evenly along one of the long edges of the stack.

9. Roll from the filled end to the unfilled end, making sure the seam-side faces down.

10. Transfer the roll to the greased sheet tray seam-side down and brush with the remaining butter.

11. In a small bowl, mix the remaining sugar and cinnamon.

12. Sprinkle it over the top and sides of the strudel.

13. Bake on the middle rack until lightly toasted or golden brown, about 12–15 minutes.

14. Remove the tray from the oven and allow the toasted strudel to rest for 5–10 minutes before slicing with a sharp knife, allowing the center to settle.

Serve.

Orange and Cinnamon Biscotti

Preparation time

1 hour 30 minutes

Ingredients

- 1 cup sugar

- ½ cup unsalted butter, room temperature

* 2 large eggs

* 2 teaspoons grated orange peel

* 1 teaspoon vanilla extract

* 2 cups all purpose flour

* 1 teaspoon cream of tartar

* ½ teaspoon baking soda

* 1 teaspoon ground cinnamon

* ¼ teaspoon salt

Instructions

1. Preheat oven to 325° F.

2. Spray 2 baking sheets with nonstick cooking spray.

3. Beat sugar and unsalted butter in a large bowl until well blended.

4. Add eggs one at a time, beating well after each.

5. Beat in orange peel and vanilla.

6. Mix flour, cream of tartar, baking soda, cinnamon and salt in a medium-size bowl.

7. Add dry ingredients to butter mixture and mix until incorporated.

8. Divide dough in half.

9. Place each half on a prepared sheet.

10. With lightly floured hands, form each half into a log shape that is 3 inches wide by three quarters of an inch high.

11. Bake until dough logs are firm to the touch, about 35 minutes.

12. Remove dough logs from oven and cool 10 minutes.

13. Transfer logs to work surface. Using serrated knife, cut on diagonal into ½-inch-thick slices.

14. Arrange cut side down on baking sheets.

15. Bake until bottoms are golden, about 12 minutes.

16. Turn biscotti over; bake until bottoms are golden, about 12 minutes longer.

17. Transfer to a wire rack and cool before serving.

www.ingramcontent.com/pod-product-compliance
Lightning Source LLC
Chambersburg PA
CBHW052016150726
47999CB00004B/1680